Nut Allergy

A Beginner's Guide to Tree Nut and Peanut Allergies, with Safe Recipes & Practical Tips

mf

copyright © 2025 Isadora Kwon

All rights reserved No part of this book may be reproduced, or stored in a retrieval system, or transmitted in any form or by any means, electronic, mechanical, photocopying, recording, or otherwise, without express written permission of the publisher.

Disclaimer

By reading this disclaimer, you are accepting the terms of the disclaimer in full. If you disagree with this disclaimer, please do not read the guide.

All of the content within this guide is provided for informational and educational purposes only, and should not be accepted as independent medical or other professional advice. The author is not a doctor, physician, nurse, mental health provider, or registered nutritionist/dietician. Therefore, using and reading this guide does not establish any form of a physician-patient relationship.

Always consult with a physician or another qualified health provider with any issues or questions you might have regarding any sort of medical condition. Do not ever disregard any qualified professional medical advice or delay seeking that advice because of anything you have read in this guide. The information in this guide is not intended to be any sort of medical advice and should not be used in lieu of any medical advice by a licensed and qualified medical professional.

The information in this guide has been compiled from a variety of known sources. However, the author cannot attest to or guarantee the accuracy of each source and thus should not be held liable for any errors or omissions.

You acknowledge that the publisher of this guide will not be held liable for any loss or damage of any kind incurred as a result of this guide or the reliance on any information provided within this guide. You acknowledge and agree that you assume all risk and responsibility for any action you undertake in response to the information in this guide.

Using this guide does not guarantee any particular result (e.g., weight loss or a cure). By reading this guide, you acknowledge that there are no guarantees to any specific outcome or results you can expect.

All product names, diet plans, or names used in this guide are for identification purposes only and are the property of their respective owners. The use of these names does not imply endorsement. All other trademarks cited herein are the property of their respective owners.

Where applicable, this guide is not intended to be a substitute for the original work of this diet plan and is, at most, a supplement to the original work for this diet plan and never a direct substitute. This guide is a personal expression of the facts of that diet plan.

Where applicable, persons shown in the cover images are stock photography models and the publisher has obtained the rights to use the images through license agreements with third-party stock image companies.

Table of Contents

Introduction   7
What Is Nut Allergy?   9
   How the Immune System Reacts to Nuts   9
   Difference Between Food Intolerance and True Allergy   11
   Types of Nut Allergies   11
Understanding Nut Allergies and Related Challenges   15
   Cross-Reactivity Between Nuts and Other Foods   15
   What Is Cross-Reactivity?   15
   Oral Allergy Syndrome (OAS) and Pollen-Food Syndrome   16
   Common Cross-Reactive Foods and Pollens   18
   Hidden Sources of Nut Allergens   18
   Who Is at Risk?   22
Causes, Symptoms, and Diagnosis   29
   How Nut Allergies Develop   29
   Common Symptoms (Mild to Severe)   30
   Allergy Testing (Skin, Blood, Oral Challenge)   32
   Which Test Is Right for You?   34
Emergency Preparedness & Treatment   35
   Recognizing Anaphylaxis   35
   Using an Epinephrine Auto-Injector (EpiPen)   40
   When to Seek Immediate Medical Help   45
Living Safely with a Nut Allergy   49
   Reading Food Labels & Identifying Hidden Nuts   49
   Avoiding Cross-Contamination   55
   Dining Out & Traveling Tips   56
Nut-Free Diet & Alternatives   63
   Safe Snack & Meal Options   63
   Cooking & Baking Without Nuts   64
   Nutrition Considerations & Substitutes   65

Nut-Free Sample Recipes   67
- Breakfast   68
- Oat-Free Energy Bowl   68
- Nut-Free Granola   69
- Sweet Potato Hash with Eggs   71
- Nut-Free Smoothie   72
- Coconut Chia Pudding   73
- Lunch & Dinner   74
- Allergy-Friendly Stir-Fry   74
- Chicken & Veggie Wraps   76
- Lentil & Quinoa Salad   77
- Potato & Leek Soup   78
- Turkey Meatballs with Rice   79
- Snacks & Desserts   80
- Sunflower Seed Butter Cookies   80
- Coconut Rice Pudding   81
- Apple Chips   82
- Frozen Yogurt Bark   83
- Dairy-Free Chocolate Mousse   84

Nut Allergies in Children & Social Settings   85
- Managing Allergies in Schools & Daycare   85
- Communicating with Caregivers & Friends   86
- Handling Social Situations & Anxiety   87

Conclusion   90
FAQs   92
References and Helpful Links   94

Introduction

Nut allergies are one of the most common food allergies, affecting millions of people around the world. These allergies occur when the immune system reacts to proteins found in certain nuts, such as peanuts or tree nuts like almonds, walnuts, and cashews. Even a small amount of these proteins can trigger allergic reactions in some individuals. These reactions vary in severity, ranging from mild symptoms like itching or hives to more serious effects, such as difficulty breathing or anaphylaxis.

The prevalence of nut allergies seems to have increased over the years, particularly among children. Research indicates that millions of people worldwide deal with these allergies, with cases often being diagnosed in early childhood. However, nut allergies can also develop later in life. Experts have studied this rise closely, though the exact reasons remain unclear. Changes in dietary habits, genetic factors, and environmental influences are some areas researchers examine.

Nut allergies require attention because they can have significant impacts on daily life. People with these allergies often need to carefully check food labels, avoid certain dishes, and stay prepared for potential allergic reactions.

Even trace amounts of nut proteins in food can pose risks for some individuals. Understanding nut allergies is not only important for those affected but also for others, including friends, family, and caregivers who prepare meals or share spaces with someone who has an allergy.

In this guide, we will talk about the following:

- What is Nut Allergy?
- Difference Between Food Intolerance and True Allergy
- Hidden Sources of Nut Allergens
- Who is at Risk?
- Causes, Symptoms, and Diagnosis
- Recognizing Anaphylaxis
- Using an Epinephrine Auto-Injector (EpiPen)
- Living Safely with a Nut Allergy
- Nut-Free Diet & Alternatives
- Nut-Free Sample Recipes
- Nut Allergies in Children & Social Settings

Keep reading to learn more about nut allergies and how you can manage them for a safe, healthy lifestyle. By the end, you will have a better understanding of nut allergies and the tools to navigate them confidently.

What Is Nut Allergy?

A nut allergy happens when a person's immune system identifies the proteins in nuts as harmful, even though they are not. This misidentification triggers an immune response. Nut allergies can involve peanuts, which are legumes, or tree nuts, like almonds, walnuts, cashews, and hazelnuts.

Even exposure to tiny amounts or traces of nuts in food can lead to a reaction for some individuals. Nut allergies can start in childhood and may persist into adulthood or develop later in life.

The symptoms range widely. Some people experience mild itching or swelling, while others may face life-threatening reactions like anaphylaxis, which requires immediate attention. The severity of symptoms often varies from person to person.

How the Immune System Reacts to Nuts

The immune system is the body's defense mechanism, designed to protect it from harmful invaders like bacteria, viruses, and other pathogens. It recognizes these threats and mounts a response to keep the body safe. However, in the case of a nut allergy, the immune system misidentifies nut proteins as harmful invaders, even though they are harmless to most people.

When someone with a nut allergy consumes or, in some cases, even comes into contact with nuts, their immune system goes into overdrive. It **produces antibodies called Immunoglobulin E (IgE)** specifically targeted at the nut proteins. These antibodies then signal the body to release chemicals, such as histamine, into the bloodstream.

This cascade of reactions results in allergy symptoms, which can vary widely in severity. Common symptoms include skin reactions like hives or rashes, swelling, difficulty breathing, a runny nose, watery eyes, and digestive issues such as nausea, vomiting, or abdominal pain.

Nut allergies are unpredictable and potentially life-threatening. Even trace amounts can trigger an immune response, and severe cases can lead to anaphylaxis, requiring immediate medical attention. This makes nut allergies particularly dangerous, emphasizing the need for strict avoidance and careful label reading. Understanding the immune reaction highlights the importance of awareness, diagnosis, and timely treatment.

Difference Between Food Intolerance and True Allergy

It is crucial to distinguish a food allergy from a food intolerance. A nut allergy involves the immune system and can cause serious, even life-threatening, symptoms. On the other hand, food intolerance does not involve the immune system and is generally less severe.

For example, someone with a nut intolerance might experience stomach discomfort, bloating, or gas after eating nuts. This occurs because their body struggles to digest certain substances in the food, not because their immune system reacts.

Allergies and intolerances may both cause discomfort, but their risks and outcomes differ greatly. Understanding this distinction highlights why nut allergies need specific care. Learning about nut allergies helps explain how the body reacts to triggers, building awareness in homes, schools, and beyond.

Types of Nut Allergies

Nut allergies can be broadly categorized into two main types: tree nut allergies and peanut allergies. While they may elicit similar allergic reactions, they are distinct in biological origin and classification, with notable differences in the foods involved.

Tree Nut Allergy

Tree nut allergies occur when the immune system reacts to proteins in nuts like almonds, walnuts, and cashews, mistaking them as harmful. Even small amounts can trigger symptoms ranging from hives and swelling to severe reactions like anaphylaxis.

Examples of Tree Nuts

Here are some commonly allergenic tree nuts:

- Almonds
- Cashews
- Walnuts
- Hazelnuts
- Pecans
- Pistachios
- Brazil Nuts
- Macadamia Nuts

Cross-Reactivity Among Tree Nuts

Tree nut allergies often involve cross-reactivity, where similar proteins in different nuts trigger allergic reactions. For example, cashew allergies may also include pistachios, and walnut allergies may involve pecans. However, sensitivities vary—some people react to only a few types, while others must avoid all tree nuts.

Peanut Allergy

Peanut allergies, by contrast, involve a reaction to peanuts, which are not biologically classified as nuts but rather as legumes. Peanuts, like lentils, chickpeas, and soybeans, grow underground and belong to the legume family. Despite being unrelated to tree nuts from a botanical and structural perspective, peanuts can trigger allergic reactions that are similar in severity to those caused by tree nuts.

Why Peanut Allergy Differs from Tree Nut Allergy

Although both trigger an allergic response, peanut and tree nut allergies are distinct for several reasons:

- *Biological Difference:* Peanuts are legumes, while tree nuts are seeds of tree-grown fruit.
- *Overlapping Allergies:* While approximately 30-40% of individuals with peanut allergies may also be allergic to tree nuts, they are often sensitized to different proteins in these distinct foods.
- *Protein Structure:* The immune system reacts to specific proteins in each food. While these proteins may cause similar symptoms, they are not identical, leading to differing patterns of allergic responses.

Peanut allergies are a major cause of severe allergic reactions and often persist into adulthood. Even trace exposure can trigger symptoms. While peanut and tree nut allergies differ biologically, both require careful management and awareness for proper diagnosis and safety.

Understanding Nut Allergies and Related Challenges

Nut allergies are already tricky to manage, but there are additional challenges that allergic individuals often face. Issues like cross-reactivity between nuts and other foods, oral allergy syndrome, and hidden sources of nut allergens can make things even more complicated. Let's break down these topics to better understand them.

Cross-Reactivity Between Nuts and Other Foods

Cross-reactivity occurs when the immune system recognizes similar proteins in different foods or substances, leading to allergic reactions across seemingly unrelated items. For individuals with nut allergies, understanding cross-reactivity is essential as it can influence how their bodies react to other foods or allergens. This phenomenon often manifests in people who experience allergic responses to both nuts and certain fruits, seeds, or pollens.

What Is Cross-Reactivity?

The immune system uses antibodies to identify and react to specific proteins, known as allergens. When two or more substances share similar structures in their proteins, the immune system may mistakenly recognize both as harmful, causing a reaction. Cross-reactivity is particularly common in food allergies, and for nut-allergic individuals, it may extend to other categories like seeds, legumes, and even pollens.

For example, a person with a tree nut allergy may also react to seeds such as sesame or sunflower due to similar protein structures. Similarly, individuals with peanut allergies may experience cross-reactions with soy or lupin, which belong to the legume family.

Oral Allergy Syndrome (OAS) and Pollen-Food Syndrome

Oral Allergy Syndrome (OAS), often referred to as Pollen-Food Syndrome, is a type of cross-reactivity where individuals allergic to certain pollen types experience allergic symptoms when consuming related foods. This is because the immune system confuses proteins in some foods with the proteins in allergenic pollens. While OAS is generally mild compared to other food allergic reactions, it often produces symptoms localized to the mouth and throat.

Connection Between Pollen Allergies and Food Reactions

OAS is a form of pollen-food cross-reactivity. People with seasonal allergies (hay fever) caused by pollen may react to fruits, vegetables, or nuts that contain structurally similar allergenic proteins. When nuts are involved, these proteins can trigger itching, tingling, or swelling in the mouth, lips, tongue, or throat, typically immediately after ingestion.

For instance:

- **Birch Pollen:** Individuals allergic to birch pollen may react to almonds, hazelnuts, and other tree nuts, as well as apples, carrots, and celery.
- **Ragweed Pollen:** Those with ragweed allergies might experience symptoms when eating melon, zucchini, or seeds, though nuts are less frequently involved.
- **Grass Pollen:** Reactions to foods like peanuts or tree nuts are less common but not unheard of in individuals sensitized to grass pollens.

Symptoms of OAS

Common symptoms of OAS include:

- Itchy or tingling sensation in the mouth or throat
- Mild swelling of the lips, tongue, or roof of the mouth
- Rarely, more severe symptoms like difficulty swallowing or difficulty breathing

Most OAS symptoms are mild and resolve quickly without the need for medication. However, more severe reactions can occur, especially in highly sensitive individuals or those with a pre-existing nut allergy.

Common Cross-Reactive Foods and Pollens

Below is a list of some of the common pollen-food cross-reactions involving nuts and other foods:

- **Birch Pollen:** Almonds, hazelnuts, cherries, apples, pears, carrots, and celery
- **Ragweed Pollen:** Melon, cucumber, zucchini, sunflower seeds
- **Grass Pollen:** Peanuts, beans, lentils (less common)
- Mugwort Pollen: Spices, such as coriander, fennel, or curry

Understanding these potential cross-reactions is crucial for individuals managing nut allergies or related conditions like hay fever. While these occurrences are common, the severity and likelihood of cross-reactivity vary greatly between individuals. Effective diagnosis by an allergist is often necessary to determine exact triggers.

By recognizing the relationship between nut allergies, pollens, and other foods, individuals can better anticipate and manage potential allergic reactions.

Hidden Sources of Nut Allergens

Nut allergens can pose significant risks, even in settings where nuts do not seem to be obvious ingredients. For individuals with nut allergies, one of the biggest challenges involves identifying hidden sources of allergens that may appear in oils, additives, or as a result of cross-contamination. Understanding these hidden dangers can help reduce unexpected exposure and increase awareness of how allergens can permeate various food products and environments.

Nut Allergens in Oils

Nut-based oils are a less obvious, but potentially significant, source of nut allergens. These oils are derived from nuts such as peanuts, almonds, or hazelnuts. While they may not always carry allergenic proteins, certain oils retain traces of the proteins that trigger allergic reactions.

Key Distinctions in Nut Oils

- *Cold-Pressed, Unrefined Oils:* These oils are mechanically extracted without high heat or chemical processing. They often contain residual nut proteins, making them unsafe for individuals with nut allergies. Examples include cold-pressed peanut or almond oil.
- *Refined Oils:* Highly processed nut oils, such as refined peanut oil, undergo heat and chemical treatment that typically removes allergenic proteins. However, not all processing is consistent, and reactions may still occur in highly sensitive individuals. Refined oils are sometimes considered safer, but validation through labeling or certification is critical.
- *Hidden Use in Foods:* Nut oils are frequently featured in restaurant cooking, salad dressings, snacks, and

gourmet products. Labeling is not always explicit, so vigilance in identifying the oil source is essential.

Additives and Nut-Derived Ingredients

Food additives can also include nut allergens, often listed under unfamiliar names or as part of complex ingredient blends. These additives may be used to enhance flavor, texture, or preservation but may unintentionally expose individuals to nut proteins.

Examples of Nut-Derived Additives

- *Natural Flavorings:* Some natural flavorings or extracts have nut-based origins, such as almond extract, which is typically made from real almonds. These flavorings are commonly used in desserts, baked goods, and syrups.
- *Thickeners or Stabilizers:* Certain food thickeners or emulsifiers, such as nut-derived gums, may include proteins that pose risks.
- *Powdered Forms:* Ground nuts or nut flours are used in some pre-packaged foods to add texture or flavor. While easily overlooked, they can have serious consequences for those with nut allergies.

Reading ingredient labels carefully is necessary since additives can be listed under unfamiliar names that do not explicitly reference nuts. Similarly, some brands may not label potential allergens due to regional regulation differences, making proper identification challenging in international or imported products.

Cross-Contamination in Food Processing

Cross-contamination is a common and avoidable hazard in food production, preparation, and handling. It refers to the unintentional transfer of allergens, including nut proteins, from one food product to another. Even when nuts are not an ingredient, exposure during manufacturing or preparation can lead to contamination.

Common Points of Nut Allergen Cross-Contamination

- *Shared Equipment:* Factories that process multiple types of food often use the same machinery for nut-based and nut-free products. While some manufacturers clean equipment between production runs, traces of nut proteins may remain.
- *Bakeries and Restaurants:* The use of shared utensils, surfaces, and cooking oils in bakeries or fast-food outlets is a frequent source of cross-contamination. For instance, baking pans may be used for both nut-based and nut-free items.
- *Bulk Bins:* Grocery store bulk bins for grains, seeds, or snacks can expose nut-free items to nut residues through shared scoops or accidental mixing.
- *Airborne Contamination:* During processing, airborne particles from nuts can settle on otherwise nut-free

foods, especially in facilities that handle large volumes of nut products.

Product Labeling and Cross-Contamination

To address these risks, some manufacturers include precautionary statements like "may contain nuts" or "produced in a facility that also processes nuts." While these labels highlight the presence of potential risks, they are voluntary in many regions and may not appear consistently.

The presence of nut allergens in oils, additives, and through cross-contamination demonstrates the importance of careful vigilance. Due to the invisible nature of some hidden sources, individuals with nut allergies and their caregivers must rely on clear labeling, transparent manufacturing processes, and detailed ingredient information to assess risk.

The scope of hidden allergens reminds us of the complexity of managing food allergies across diverse food and cooking environments. Recognizing these potential exposures helps increase awareness and fosters safer practices for individuals living with nut allergies.

Who Is at Risk?

Nut allergies are a prevalent food allergy, impacting people of all ages and backgrounds. However, not everyone shares the same level of risk for developing nut allergies. A combination of genetic predisposition, environmental exposure, and age-related factors determines the likelihood of having a nut allergy.

This section explores the different influences—ranging from hereditary tendencies to why allergies might emerge later in life—and provides insights into how these factors interplay.

Genetic & Environmental Factors

1. *The Role of Genetics*

   Genetics play a major role in determining whether an individual is likely to develop a nut allergy. If one or both parents have a history of allergies, including food allergies, eczema, hay fever, or asthma, their children are more likely to inherit similar conditions. This pattern indicates how susceptibility to allergies often runs in families.

   For nut allergies specifically, certain genetic markers influence how the immune system responds to allergens. These markers can predispose individuals to having a hyperactive immune response to typically harmless nut proteins. Additionally, siblings of people with nut allergies are at an increased risk, underlining the significance of familial influence.

2. *Environmental Influences*

   Environmental factors also contribute significantly to the likelihood of developing nut allergies. The timing, frequency, and manner of exposure to nuts during early life are key considerations:

- ***Dietary Exposure:*** Delayed introduction of allergenic foods like nuts during infancy has been associated with an increased risk of developing allergies. Studies suggest that early and controlled exposure may help the immune system develop tolerance.
- ***Lifestyle Considerations:*** Children raised in more urbanized settings tend to have higher allergy rates compared to those in rural environments. This "hygiene hypothesis" suggests that reduced early exposure to diverse microbes limits immune system development and increases the risk of allergies.
- ***Environmental Allergens and Pollution:*** Pollution and exposure to allergens in the environment, such as pollen or dust mites, may prime the immune system, making it more susceptible to food allergies, including nut allergies.

The interplay of genetic predisposition and environmental exposure shapes individual outcomes, explaining why some people are more vulnerable to developing nut allergies than others.

Nut Allergies in Children vs. Adults

Nut Allergies in Children

Nut allergies are most common in children and often become apparent during early childhood. Symptoms typically develop within minutes to hours after consuming nuts and can range from mild reactions, such as hives, to severe symptoms, including anaphylaxis. Children with other allergic conditions, such as eczema or asthma, are at greater risk of having nut allergies.

For many children, nut allergies tend to be lifelong. Unlike some other food allergies—such as milk or egg allergies—that children can outgrow with age, nut allergies have a significantly lower outgrowth rate. Studies estimate that only about 10-20% of children with tree nut or peanut allergies will eventually outgrow them.

Nut Allergies in Adults

While most nut allergies first appear in childhood, allergies can persist into adulthood or even develop later in life. Adults with nut allergies may experience unpredictable or severe allergic responses, particularly since they may be unaware of their allergy until the first reaction occurs.

Some adults experience a phenomenon known as lipid transfer protein (LTP) syndrome, where cross-reactivity occurs between specific nut proteins and other plant-based foods like certain fruits or seeds. This can lead to a broadening of allergic symptoms over time.

Severity Differences Between Age Groups

The prevalence of nut allergies is higher in children than in adults, but the severity of reactions does not necessarily decrease with age. Children are often more vulnerable to accidental exposure, particularly in school environments where they have less control over food preparation.

Education and awareness about managing allergies tend to improve in adulthood, potentially reducing the risk of accidental exposure in adult patients.

Why Some Allergies Develop Later in Life

Not all allergies develop in childhood. Some people may experience their first allergic reaction to nuts well into adulthood. This delayed onset raises questions about why some individuals develop nut allergies later in life despite a prior absence of symptoms.

1. *Immune System Changes*

   Over time, the immune system undergoes changes that can affect the way the body responds to allergens. Certain life events or illnesses can increase immune sensitivity. These include:

- **Major Illness or Infection:** Severe illnesses or infections can disrupt immune system balance, triggering abnormal immune responses to previously tolerated foods like nuts.
- **Hormonal Changes:** Factors such as pregnancy, menopause, or hormonal shifts may also influence immune system function and create new sensitivities.

2. *Lifestyle and Exposure*

Changes in lifestyle or dietary habits later in life may increase exposure to nuts or nut-derived ingredients, triggering an allergy in otherwise unaffected individuals. For example, a change in diet that heavily incorporates nut-based products could increase the likelihood of sensitization to nut proteins.

3. *Cross-Reactivity*

Another explanation for adult-onset nut allergies is cross-reactivity. Cross-reactivity happens when the immune system mistakes proteins in nuts for similar proteins found in other substances.

For instance, individuals with pollen allergies may suddenly develop sensitivity to nuts due to this immune misidentification, resulting in a phenomenon known as oral allergy syndrome (OAS).

4. *Diminished Tolerance*

Tolerance to allergens can also diminish over time. An individual who previously consumed nuts without issue may lose their tolerance due to long intervals of avoidance or other unknown factors. This loss of tolerance can lead to an unexpected allergic response upon re-exposure.

Understanding who is at risk for nut allergies involves examining the complex relationship between genetic tendencies, environmental influences, age, and immune system changes. While genetics and early exposures play significant roles in childhood development of nut allergies, adults are not exempt from developing such sensitivities later in life.

By exploring these risk factors, we gain a clearer picture of why nut allergies affect certain individuals differently and the ongoing challenges faced by those living with them.

Causes, Symptoms, and Diagnosis

Nut allergies are among the most common food allergies, affecting both children and adults. Understanding how these allergies develop, recognizing the range of symptoms, and knowing how they are diagnosed can help individuals manage them effectively. Here's a breakdown of the causes, symptoms, and testing methods behind nut allergies.

How Nut Allergies Develop

Nut allergies occur when the immune system mistakes certain nut proteins as harmful substances. Normally, the immune system works to fight off things like bacteria or viruses. But in people with nut allergies, it misidentifies these proteins and reacts as if they're a threat.

This response results in the release of chemicals like histamine, which causes allergic symptoms. The exact reason why some people develop nut allergies isn't fully understood, but several factors play a role:

- *Genetics:* If allergies, asthma, or eczema run in your family, you're more likely to have a nut allergy.

- *Age:* Nut allergies often begin in childhood, but they can develop at any age.
- *Exposure:* Some research suggests early exposure to nuts may either increase or decrease the risk, depending on individual factors.
- *Immune Sensitivity:* People with other allergies or sensitive immune systems may be more prone to developing new ones, like nut allergies.

Once a nut allergy develops, it often persists throughout life, although a small percentage of children with nut allergies may outgrow them.

Common Symptoms (Mild to Severe)

The symptoms of nut allergies vary widely in intensity. For some individuals, reactions are mild and manageable, but for others, exposure to nuts can cause a severe, life-threatening condition known as anaphylaxis. Identifying the symptoms promptly is essential to managing the allergy safely.

Mild Symptoms

Mild reactions are often limited to one part of the body and are typically short-lived. Examples include:

- *Skin Rash or Hives:* Red, itchy, raised welts that can appear anywhere on the body.
- *Itchy Mouth or Throat:* A tingling or itchy sensation, particularly after eating nuts.

- *Mild Digestive Distress:* Symptoms like stomach discomfort, mild cramping, or nausea may occur.

Moderate Symptoms

A moderate reaction can involve multiple systems in the body and may require medical attention. Common symptoms include:

- *Swelling:* Puffiness, particularly around the lips, eyes, or face.
- *Respiratory Symptoms:* Congestion, wheezing, coughing, or shortness of breath caused by swelling of the respiratory passages.
- *Vomiting or Diarrhea:* These symptoms may appear shortly after consuming nuts and signal a more systemic reaction.

Severe Symptoms (Anaphylaxis)

Severe reactions, known as anaphylaxis, are medical emergencies requiring immediate treatment. Symptoms can affect multiple organ systems and escalate rapidly. Severe signs include:

- *Difficulty Breathing:* Swelling of the throat, tongue, or airways can cause wheezing or restricted breathing.
- *Drop in Blood Pressure (Shock):* This can lead to dizziness, fainting, or loss of consciousness.

- ***Rapid Swelling:*** Extensive swelling that contributes to airway obstruction and other complications.

Anaphylaxis can occur within minutes of exposure and can lead to severe complications or death without medical intervention.

Allergy Testing (Skin, Blood, Oral Challenge)

Correctly diagnosing nut allergies is crucial to managing the condition effectively. This requires professional assessment through a variety of tests designed to confirm an immune response to nut proteins and determine the severity of the allergy. The following are the most common diagnostic methods used by allergists.

Skin Test

The skin prick test is one of the most widely used tools for diagnosing nut allergies. During this procedure:

1. A small amount of nut protein extract is placed on the surface of the skin, usually on the forearm or back.
2. The skin is lightly pricked to allow the extract to enter the top layer.
3. If the individual is allergic, a raised, itchy bump (similar to a mosquito bite) will appear within 15–20 minutes at the test site.

While the skin test is effective at identifying IgE-mediated allergies, it is not suitable for individuals with severe allergies where exposure may cause an adverse reaction.

Blood Test

Blood testing measures the levels of specific IgE antibodies in the bloodstream to determine sensitivity to nuts. This test involves:

1. Drawing a blood sample.
2. Analyzing the sample in a laboratory to detect the presence and quantity of nut-specific IgE antibodies.

Blood tests are particularly useful when a skin test is not advisable—such as when a patient has a skin condition or requires medications that might interfere with the results. However, it's worth noting that blood tests may produce false positives, and results are typically interpreted alongside other clinical evidence.

Oral Food Challenge

The oral challenge test is considered the most definitive way to diagnose a nut allergy. It is usually conducted in a controlled medical environment to ensure safety. The procedure involves:

1. Administering small but increasing amounts of the suspected allergenic food (e.g., nuts) under close supervision.

2. Monitoring for symptoms or reactions at each stage.

If the individual exhibits an allergic response, the test is stopped immediately, and appropriate treatment is administered. Oral food challenges are typically reserved for cases where other tests yield inconclusive results or for assessing whether a child has outgrown their allergy.

Which Test Is Right for You?

Your healthcare provider will recommend the best test based on your symptoms, history, and overall health. Sometimes, a combination of tests is used to make a clear diagnosis.

Understanding nut allergies, recognizing symptoms, and getting proper diagnostic tests are key to managing the condition. Early identification, whether symptoms are mild or severe, helps you stay safe. If you suspect a nut allergy, consult an allergist to find the right solution for you.

Emergency Preparedness & Treatment

Dealing with severe allergic reactions, like those caused by nut allergies, can be scary. Knowing what to do in an emergency can make all the difference. This chapter will walk you through how to recognize anaphylaxis, the correct way to use an epinephrine auto-injector (commonly called an EpiPen), and when to get professional medical help.

Recognizing Anaphylaxis

Anaphylaxis is one of the most severe and alarming allergic reactions a person can experience. It is characterized by a rapid onset and potentially life-threatening symptoms, making it a medical emergency that requires immediate attention. For individuals with allergies, such as nut allergies, understanding the signs, how they develop, and the risks involved is essential to ensuring safety and timely intervention.

What Is Anaphylaxis?

Anaphylaxis is a systemic allergic reaction that occurs when the body's immune system overreacts to a substance it mistakenly identifies as harmful. This systemic reaction creates a cascade of events in the body, including the sudden release of chemical mediators like histamine.

These substances cause widespread inflammation, which can disrupt multiple organ systems, including the respiratory, cardiovascular, and gastrointestinal systems. Unlike mild allergic reactions, anaphylaxis can impair breathing, cause a dangerous drop in blood pressure, and lead to severe complications or even death if left untreated.

How Does It Develop?

Anaphylaxis is triggered by exposure to an allergen. For individuals with food allergies, nuts (both tree nuts and peanuts) are a common cause. When the immune system identifies the allergen, antibodies called Immunoglobulin E (IgE) bind to it. This sets off a massive immune response, including the activation of mast cells and basophils, which release chemicals like histamine into the bloodstream.

The release of these substances leads to the symptoms associated with anaphylaxis, such as swelling, difficulty breathing, and cardiovascular collapse. It is the systemic nature of the reaction—affecting multiple parts of the body at once—that makes anaphylaxis so dangerous.

Recognizing Symptoms of Anaphylaxis

The symptoms of anaphylaxis can vary in presentation and severity, but they often escalate rapidly. Recognizing these symptoms early is vital because delaying treatment increases the risk of life-threatening complications. Symptoms can affect the skin, respiratory system, cardiovascular system, and gastrointestinal tract.

Common Symptoms

1. ***Swelling:*** Swelling is one of the hallmark symptoms of anaphylaxis and can occur in various parts of the body. Swelling of the face, lips, tongue, or throat is particularly concerning because it can block airways, making it difficult or impossible to breathe.
2. ***Difficulty Breathing or Wheezing:*** Constriction of the airways caused by swelling or inflammation in the respiratory system can lead to labored breathing or wheezing. This is often coupled with a sensation of tightness in the chest, making breathing increasingly difficult as the reaction progresses.
3. ***Chest Tightness or Pain:*** Chest tightness may be due to airway constriction or cardiovascular strain. Pain or discomfort in the chest can be an early warning of respiratory or circulatory distress, both of which are serious complications of anaphylaxis.
4. ***Cardiovascular Symptoms:*** A rapid heartbeat (tachycardia) or a sudden drop in blood pressure

(hypotension) is a common feature of anaphylaxis. When blood pressure drops, it can lead to dizziness, fainting, or shock—a state where the body's vital organs do not receive enough blood flow.
5. ***Skin Symptoms:*** Severe, widespread hives or rash are common during anaphylaxis. The skin may become flushed, red, and intensely itchy. These symptoms often appear quickly after exposure to the allergen.
6. ***Gastrointestinal Symptoms:*** Nausea, vomiting, diarrhea, and abdominal cramping often accompany anaphylaxis, particularly in food-related reactions. These symptoms can worsen rapidly, further straining the body during the allergic response.
7. ***Neurological Symptoms:*** Some people experiencing anaphylaxis report a sudden feeling of doom or intense confusion. This psychological symptom arises from the panic and physical strain caused by the reaction.

It's important to note that symptoms do not always present themselves in a predictable order, and they can develop differently in each individual. For some, mild symptoms, such as a runny nose or stomach upset, may precede more severe signs like difficulty breathing or sudden collapse. For others, severe symptoms may appear almost immediately after exposure.

Why Immediate Treatment Is Critical

Time is a critical factor in managing anaphylaxis. The condition can escalate from mild to severe in just minutes and may lead to fatal complications if untreated. The release of inflammatory chemicals can cause airway obstruction, heart failure, or profound hypotension—all of which can occur suddenly without warning. Early recognition allows for quicker intervention, which can prevent severe outcomes.

Intervention is typically aimed at counteracting the allergic reaction and stabilizing the body's systems. Delayed treatment increases the likelihood of complications such as hypoxic brain injury, prolonged shock, or organ failure.

Factors That May Delay Treatment

- ***Uncertainty About Symptoms:*** Symptoms overlap with other conditions, like asthma or panic attacks, which may lead to hesitation in recognizing anaphylaxis.
- ***Mild Initial Symptoms:*** Some cases begin with mild symptoms that may seem harmless, causing individuals to delay seeking help.
- ***Lack of Awareness:*** Not recognizing anaphylaxis as an emergency can lead to delayed action, increasing risks.

Anaphylaxis is a condition where minutes matter. Even if you're unsure whether someone is experiencing anaphylaxis, treating it as such is safer than waiting to see if symptoms worsen. Immediate action can prevent severe complications and potentially save a life. It is better to err on the side of caution and seek medical attention at the first sign of a severe allergic reaction.

Using an Epinephrine Auto-Injector (EpiPen)

An epinephrine auto-injector, commonly referred to by brand names like EpiPen, is a life-saving device designed to deliver a precise dose of epinephrine during a severe allergic reaction, also known as anaphylaxis.

For individuals with serious allergies, having access to and knowing how to use an epinephrine auto-injector can mean the difference between life and death. This section provides an overview of what the device is, how it works, and how to use it effectively in an emergency.

During anaphylaxis, administering epinephrine can:

- **Reduce throat and airway swelling** to restore breathing.
- **Increase blood pressure** when it has dropped due to vasodilation (dilated blood vessels).
- **Counteract histamine release** to mitigate symptoms like hives or swelling.
- **Improve cardiovascular function** by increasing heart rate and output.

Epinephrine acts rapidly to stabilize the body, buying critical time until additional medical treatment is available. It is the first-line treatment for anaphylaxis and is preferred over other medications, such as antihistamines, which act too slowly to be effective in severe allergic reactions.

How an Epinephrine Auto-Injector Works

The auto-injector is designed to be easy to operate, even during high-stress situations:

- It contains a spring-loaded needle that automatically releases when the device is activated.
- Once pressed against the skin, the needle administers the medication directly into the outer thigh muscle, where it is absorbed into the bloodstream within minutes.
- This rapid delivery ensures the medication starts working against the life-threatening symptoms of anaphylaxis almost immediately.

Most epinephrine auto-injectors are single-use devices. After using one, medical attention should still be sought, as symptoms may recur or require further stabilization.

When to Use an Epinephrine Auto-Injector

An epinephrine auto-injector should be administered at the first sign of suspected anaphylaxis. **Immediate use is critical if any of the following symptoms are observed**:

- Rapid swelling of the throat, tongue, or face.
- Difficulty breathing, wheezing, or choking sensations.
- A sudden drop in blood pressure causing dizziness, fainting, or confusion.
- Severe hives or rash that spread rapidly across the body.
- Persistent nausea, vomiting, or diarrhea accompanied by other symptoms of anaphylaxis.

Because anaphylaxis can escalate quickly, waiting to see if symptoms worsen is not safe. Administering the auto-injector immediately after symptoms appear can prevent the reaction from becoming more severe.

Step-by-Step Instructions for Using an Epinephrine Auto-Injector

Knowing how to use an epinephrine auto-injector beforehand can help ensure quick and effective action during an emergency. While specific devices may vary slightly in operation, the general steps are outlined below:

1. ***Position the Device Correctly:***
   - Hold the auto-injector firmly, keeping your fingers away from both ends.
   - Identify the tip containing the needle and aim this side downward. Most auto-injectors are clearly labeled or color-coded for ease of identification.

2. ***Remove the Safety Cap:*** Pull off the safety cap to activate the injector. This prepares the device for use.
3. ***Administer the Injection:***
   - Place the tip of the auto-injector against the outer thigh. Injection through clothing is safe and effective, so there's no need to remove pants or other barriers.
   - Press the device firmly into the thigh until you hear a click, which signifies the needle has been deployed and the medication is being injected.
   - Hold the injector in place for 5–10 seconds to ensure the full dose is delivered.
4. ***Withdraw the Injector:*** Remove the injector and safely dispose of the used device, following local medical waste guidelines or placing it into its protective case. The needle will automatically retract in most devices to prevent accidental pricks.
5. ***Monitor the Individual:*** While waiting for emergency responders, monitor the person's condition closely. Lay them flat on their back unless breathing is difficult, in which case they should be propped up. Avoid giving them food or drink.

Even after the symptoms improve, you must seek immediate medical attention. Further treatment may be necessary as anaphylaxis symptoms can return (known as a biphasic reaction) within hours.

How to Store an Epinephrine Auto-Injector

Proper storage ensures the device will function effectively when needed:

- *Store at Room Temperature:* Avoid exposing the auto-injector to extreme temperatures. Epinephrine can degrade if stored in excessively hot or cold conditions, reducing its effectiveness.
- *Keep It Accessible:* Always carry the auto-injector with you if you have known allergies. Ensure it is stored in an easily accessible location, such as a purse, backpack, or pocket, rather than in hard-to-reach places.
- *Check the Expiration Date:* Epinephrine auto-injectors have expiration dates. Regularly check the device and replace it before it expires to ensure it delivers an effective dose during emergencies.
- *Inspect for Damage:* Inspect the injector periodically. If the liquid appears cloudy, discolored or contains particles, replace the device.

Why Epinephrine is Critical in Managing Anaphylaxis

During an anaphylactic reaction, every second matters. Epinephrine auto-injectors provide fast, life-saving intervention by quickly opening airways, restoring blood pressure, and preventing complications. Unlike antihistamines or corticosteroids, only epinephrine acts quickly enough to address the root causes of anaphylaxis.

Knowing how to use an epinephrine auto-injector is crucial for managing severe allergies and anaphylaxis. Quick action and preparation can save lives during allergic emergencies.

When to Seek Immediate Medical Help

Symptoms of allergic reactions can vary widely depending on the individual and the nature of the allergen. Some signs clearly indicate the need for emergency care. Being able to recognize these symptoms can make all the difference.

Signs That Require Immediate Emergency Care

Severe allergic reactions, like anaphylaxis, can escalate quickly and demand urgent medical care. The symptoms listed below signal a life-threatening allergic reaction and require immediate emergency assistance:

- *Breathing Difficulties:* Wheezing, choking, gasping, or outright inability to breathe due to airway swelling.
- *Swelling:* Significant swelling of the face, lips, tongue, or throat, which can obstruct airways and impact breathing or swallowing.
- *Circulatory Symptoms:* Sudden dizziness, fainting, or confusion caused by a significant drop in blood pressure (shock).
- *Rapid Progression of Symptoms:* Multiple symptoms appearing simultaneously, such as hives coupled with difficulty breathing and abdominal pain.

- **Chest Pain or Tightness:** This may be accompanied by shortness of breath or a feeling of heaviness, signaling a cardiovascular strain.
- **Severe Gastrointestinal Symptoms:** Persistent vomiting, diarrhea, or abdominal cramping that is not relieved and occurs alongside other symptoms of anaphylaxis.
- **Feeling of Doom:** A sudden, unexplained sense of impending doom or severe anxiety, often reported by individuals experiencing anaphylaxis.

When these symptoms are present, time is of the essence. Even if you are unsure about the severity, it is always safer to treat the situation as an emergency rather than waiting to see if symptoms resolve.

The Risks of Delaying Treatment

Waiting to seek medical help during an allergic reaction, especially one involving anaphylaxis, can put the individual at greater risk of severe complications, including:

- **Airway Obstruction:** Swelling in the throat or tongue can completely block the airway, making breathing impossible. Without intervention, this can lead to suffocation.
- **Cardiovascular Collapse:** Anaphylaxis can cause blood pressure to plummet, leading to shock and potentially fatal outcomes if not treated promptly.

- ***Organ Failure:*** Insufficient oxygen or blood flow to vital organs during severe allergic reactions can result in irreversible damage.
- ***Biphasic Reaction:*** Symptoms may subside temporarily, only to reappear hours later with equal or greater severity. Without professional observation and treatment, the second phase can be even more dangerous.

Medical care not only addresses the immediate danger but also ensures appropriate monitoring for delayed or lingering symptoms.

The Role of Emergency Care in Managing Allergic Reactions

Emergency medical professionals are trained to treat allergic reactions effectively and prevent complications. The primary goals of emergency care are to stabilize the individual, treat the reaction, and protect against further harm. Key treatments provided during emergency care include:

- ***Epinephrine Administration:*** Epinephrine is the first-line treatment for anaphylaxis, effectively reversing symptoms such as airway swelling, low blood pressure, and respiratory distress.
- ***Oxygen Therapy:*** For individuals struggling to breathe, supplemental oxygen ensures sufficient oxygen levels in the bloodstream.

- ***Intravenous Fluids:*** When blood pressure drops dangerously low, IV fluids help maintain circulation and prevent shock.
- ***Antihistamines and Steroids:*** These medications may be used to reduce inflammation and prevent prolonged symptoms after the immediate reaction is controlled.

Additionally, emergency care providers monitor individuals for biphasic reactions or other complications, ensuring they remain stable before being discharged or transferred to continued care.

Knowing when to seek medical help during an allergic reaction is crucial for minimizing risks and safeguarding health. The distinction between mild and severe symptoms guides the urgency of action, and recognizing the signs of a life-threatening reaction, such as anaphylaxis, ensures swift access to life-saving care.

Living Safely with a Nut Allergy

For individuals with nut allergies, taking steps to minimize risk is essential for safety. Everyday activities like grocery shopping, dining out, or traveling require careful attention to avoid exposure to allergens. The following sections explore key elements in managing the risks associated with nut allergies.

Reading Food Labels & Identifying Hidden Nuts

For individuals with nut allergies, reading food labels is not just a precaution—it's a vital skill to prevent severe allergic reactions. Nuts are one of the most common allergens, and even trace amounts can trigger serious or potentially life-threatening symptoms in some individuals. Despite clear labeling regulations, nuts can appear in unexpected ways, making attentiveness and knowledge essential for identifying potential risks.

This section explores why reading labels is critical, how to identify nuts and related ingredients, the implications of cross-contact warnings, and examples of hidden sources of nuts in everyday products.

Why Reading Food Labels Is Crucial

Food labels provide essential information about the contents of packaged products, including the presence of common allergens such as tree nuts and peanuts. Allergic reactions to nuts can occur even with small quantities, so accurately identifying nut-derived ingredients is necessary to avoid exposure.

Regulations in many countries require manufacturers to clearly indicate major allergens on their packaging. This helps individuals with food allergies make informed decisions and reduces the risk of accidental consumption. However, less obvious sources of nuts, ambiguous ingredient names, and variations in manufacturing processes can introduce challenges when identifying allergens.

Remaining vigilant about food labels and educating oneself on potential hidden sources of nuts ensures better safety and reduces the risks associated with accidental exposure.

Identifying Nuts on Labels

Nuts are classified as major allergens and, as such, must be clearly listed on product labels in many regions under food labeling laws. They may appear in two key ways:

1. *Ingredient Lists*

Food labels list all ingredients in descending order of quantity. When a product contains nuts, their specific type—such as almonds, pecans, walnuts, or cashews—will be named explicitly. For example:

- **Cashews** in granola bars.
- **Almonds** in baked goods.
- **Walnuts** in trail mixes or desserts.

Some products also include nut-derived ingredients such as powders, flours, or oils. These must also be labeled. For example, almond flour used in gluten-free baked goods must appear as "Almond Flour" in the ingredient list.

2. *"Contains" Statements*

Many packaged food items include an allergen summary below the ingredient list under a "Contains" statement. This section identifies any allergens explicitly used in the product. For example:

- "Contains tree nuts (hazelnuts, cashews)."
- "Contains almonds."

These statements provide extra clarity by consolidating allergen information, making it easier for consumers to verify the presence of nuts.

Warnings for Cross-Contact

Some products carry precautionary warnings such as "May contain traces of nuts." These warnings indicate the possibility of cross-contact during manufacturing. Cross-contact occurs when equipment or facilities handling nut-containing foods are also used to process other products. While nuts may not be an intended ingredient, trace amounts could inadvertently contaminate nut-free recipes.

Examples of common cross-contact warnings include:

- "May contain peanuts or tree nuts."
- "Processed in a facility that also handles tree nuts."

Cross-contact warnings are voluntary and not standardized, so the wording might differ. However, such labels serve as an alert for potential risks. Consumers with severe nut allergies should take these warnings seriously, as even trace amounts can provoke allergic reactions in sensitive individuals.

Hidden Sources of Nuts

While nuts might seem easy to identify in plain forms, they often appear in hidden or unexpected ways within packaged foods, sauces, baked goods, and beverages. Recognizing these hidden sources is key to avoiding accidental exposure.

Examples of Hidden Nut Ingredients

1. **<u>Nut-Based Ingredients Disguised by Name</u>**

Some food products contain nut-derived ingredients that are not explicitly labeled as nuts. Examples include:

- *Marzipan* (made from almonds): Commonly used in candies, pastries, or holiday confections.
- *Nougat* (may contain peanuts or almonds): Frequently found in candies and chocolate bars.
- *Pesto sauces* (traditionally made with pine nuts but often using cashews or walnuts as substitutes): Used in pasta, sandwiches, or as a topping.

2. **Nut Oils and Extracts**

Nut oils and extracts are often added to enhance flavor but might not be readily apparent as allergens:

- *Almond oil* (used in some salad dressings and beauty products).
- *Walnut oil* (used in gourmet cooking or condiments).
- *Nut extracts*, such as hazelnut extract or almond flavoring, are found in desserts, baked goods, or flavored drinks.

3. **Desserts and Candy**

Sweets are a common culprit for hidden nuts, as they often include nut fillings or coatings:

- *Chocolates and truffles* filled with hazelnut paste or almond praline.
- *Cookies, pastries, or cakes* using almond flour or ground nuts as a base.
- *Ice creams* with nut flavors or in close contact with nut-inclusive varieties during manufacturing.

4. **Savory Snacks and Seasonings**

Some savory or processed goods may also contain nuts or nut derivatives:

- Trail mixes, granola, or energy bars with "hidden" nuts beyond the obvious ones.
- Pre-seasoned dishes that incorporate nut oils or crushed nuts as garnishes or ingredients.

5. **Beverages**
   - Flavored coffees, lattes, or other beverages may include nut syrups or flavorings such as hazelnut or almond syrup.
   - Some protein shakes and non-dairy milks (e.g., cashew milk, almond milk) may contain traces of nuts even if labeled as safe alternatives.

Regularly Review Labels

Manufacturing processes and recipes can change over time. A product that was previously nut-free may later contain nuts due to updated formulations or shared equipment. For this reason, individuals with nut allergies should always review food labels—even on products they've consumed previously. Staying informed and checking for updates is an essential step in avoiding allergens.

Reading food labels and identifying hidden nuts is an indispensable practice for individuals with nut allergies. The combination of clear ingredient labeling, allergen warnings, and taking note of hidden sources allows consumers to make safer choices.

By carefully scanning labels and recognizing less obvious signs of nut content, individuals can better protect themselves against the risks of accidental exposure. Awareness and vigilance are the best defenses against the challenges posed by nut allergens in everyday products.

Avoiding Cross-Contamination

Cross-contamination occurs when a nut-containing product comes into contact with an allergen-free item, making it unsafe for individuals with nut allergies. This can happen during food preparation, handling, or storage.

- *At Home:* The risk of cross-contamination begins in the kitchen. Shared utensils, cutting boards, or appliances like blenders can transfer trace amounts of nut allergens between foods. If nut-containing products

and allergen-free items are stored closely together, the risk of transfer also increases.
- ***In Food Production:*** Factories that produce multiple food products often process nut-containing items on the same equipment used for other foods. Although some facilities clean their equipment thoroughly, traces of nut proteins may remain, posing a risk to highly sensitive individuals. Labels with "processed in the same facility" statements warn of this possibility.
- ***During Meal Preparation:*** Shared serving utensils, buffets, or salad bars can all contribute to cross-contamination risks. Even items prepared without nuts may come into contact with them through equipment or surfaces.

Being aware of the potential for cross-contamination in these contexts can help individuals assess and manage their exposure risk.

Dining Out & Traveling Tips

For individuals with nut allergies, dining out and traveling can be particularly challenging. Foods prepared in unfamiliar settings or served in different regions often come with hidden or unavoidable risks, making vigilance and preparation essential.

Risks in Restaurant Food Preparation

Restaurants are exciting places to enjoy a variety of cuisines, but they can also present heightened risks for those with nut allergies. Understanding how allergens may enter dishes during food preparation is critical to navigating this environment safely.

Nuts as Ingredients

Nuts may be used in numerous ways in restaurant settings—sometimes as obvious components and sometimes in more subtle forms:

- *Central Ingredients:* Many dishes, particularly in ethnic cuisines, feature nuts prominently. Examples include peanut-based sauces in Thai cooking, cashew gravies in Indian curries, or ground nuts in African stews.
- *Garnishes:* Nuts such as almond slivers, crushed walnuts, or pecans are often sprinkled on salads, desserts, or even main dishes for added texture and flavor.
- *Desserts and Baked Goods:* Nuts and nut butter frequently appear in pies, cookies, cakes, and pastries. Even items that do not directly list nuts as an ingredient may be cross-contaminated during baking.

Risk of Cross-Contamination

Cross-contamination occurs when non-nut dishes come into contact with nuts or nut-containing ingredients during preparation. This can happen when:

- Restaurants use the same deep fryers for multiple dishes, meaning oil used to fry nut-coated items could later be used for another dish.
- Kitchen utensils, cutting boards, or preparation spaces are not thoroughly cleaned between handling nut and non-nut ingredients.
- Nut-based toppings or garnishes (e.g., crushed peanuts) accidentally spill onto adjacent plates during service.

Even trace amounts can trigger severe allergic reactions, making cross-contamination a significant concern in restaurant environments.

Communication Strategies When Dining Out

Communicating effectively with restaurant staff is one of the most important steps for successfully managing nut allergies while eating out. Clear and early communication ensures that precautions can be taken to reduce risks.

Informing Staff About Allergies

It is crucial to notify restaurant staff of any nut allergies before ordering. Key points for communication include:

- ***Explaining the Allergy Severity:*** Specify that the allergy includes even trace amounts or cross-contamination, so the seriousness is fully understood.
- ***Clarifying Ingredients:*** Ask direct questions about whether nuts or nut oils are used in the dish or its preparation, especially for sauces, dressings, and desserts.
- ***Verifying Cooking Processes:*** Confirm whether the equipment is shared between the nut and non-nut dishes, particularly for frying or mixing ingredients.

Training and Allergy Protocols

Some restaurants are better prepared to handle food allergies due to staff training and established allergen protocols. These may include:

- Clearly marked menus or allergen guides that identify dishes safe for those with nut allergies.
- Staff who are trained to accommodate allergy requests by communicating with the kitchen directly or customizing orders.
- Specialized preparation areas in kitchens to reduce the risk of cross-contamination.

Choosing restaurants with such protocols can make dining out safer and less stressful.

Travel Considerations for Nut Allergies

Traveling presents additional challenges for those with nut allergies, whether navigating meals during flights, exploring new cuisines, or dealing with potential allergen exposure in non-food products.

Traveling by Air

Air travel poses unique risks, especially since travelers are confined to a shared space and may not have control over their food options:

- ***Airline Meals and Snacks:*** Many airlines provide snacks like peanuts or tree nuts and may include nut ingredients in pre-packaged meals. Even if nuts are not served, cross-contact with shared manufacturing facilities can occur.
- ***Allergen Residue:*** Nut residue on tray tables, seats, or armrests from previous passengers may pose a risk. Travelers with nut allergies must remain cautious about their seating environment.

Navigating International Cuisines

Certain cuisines around the world rely heavily on nuts or nut-derived ingredients, which could increase the frequency of potential exposures:

- *Asian Cuisines* such as Thai, Vietnamese, and Korean cooking often feature peanuts and cashews in sauces, stir-fries, and side dishes.
- *Middle Eastern and Mediterranean Foods* include ingredients like ground almonds, crushed pistachios, or pine nuts in both savory dishes and desserts.
- *African and Indian Cooking* may use nuts, nut oils, or nut flours in stews, gravies, or breads.

Non-Food Sources of Nuts

Nut oils and extracts can also appear in certain non-food items that travelers may encounter, such as:

- Skincare Products like lotions or creams containing almond or walnut oil.
- Regional Crafts or Gifts made from nut shells or oils.

Meal Planning and Preparation

Careful planning is essential for reducing risks while traveling:

- *Pack Snacks:* Bringing certified nut-free snacks ensures access to safe food in case options are limited during travel or in unfamiliar locations.
- *Research Local Food Options:* Understanding the common ingredients and dishes used in the destination's cuisine helps identify potential risks.

Dining out and traveling with nut allergies requires careful preparation and clear communication to manage risks like cross-contamination and hidden allergens. With proactive strategies, individuals can enjoy safer, more enjoyable experiences.

Nut-Free Diet & Alternatives

For individuals managing a nut allergy or choosing to avoid nuts, adapting to a nut-free diet involves understanding safe food options, cooking and baking adjustments, and alternative sources of essential nutrients. Below, we explore these aspects to provide clarity on maintaining a nut-free lifestyle.

Safe Snack & Meal Options

Eliminating nuts from meals and snacks can be straightforward with an understanding of allergy-safe foods. This includes both naturally nut-free items and foods processed in nut-free environments.

- **Fruits and Vegetables:** Fresh produce is naturally nut-free and widely considered safe for consumption. These can be eaten raw, cooked, or as ingredients in recipes for snacks or meals.
- **Whole Grains:** Options such as rice, oats, quinoa, and barley are nut-free and versatile for creating nutritionally balanced dishes. Examples include oatmeal, rice bowls, or grain-based salads.

- ***Protein Sources:*** Foods like eggs, fish, poultry, beans, lentils, and tofu offer alternatives to nuts as protein sources. Seeds such as sunflower or pumpkin seeds can serve as snacks or toppings in some cases, although their safety depends on manufacturing processes and any risk of cross-contamination.
- ***Packaged Foods:*** Snacks specifically labeled as "nut-free" may include products such as nut-free granola bars, crackers, or cookies. Individuals should verify labels to ensure compliance with their dietary requirements and identify potential cross-contact warnings.

Understanding food sourcing, preparation, and manufacturing is essential to ensure snacks and meals are entirely nut-free.

Cooking & Baking Without Nuts

Cooking and baking without nuts requires ingredient substitutions to maintain flavors, textures, or nutritional qualities in recipes.

- ***Flavor Substitutes:*** Roasted chickpeas, seeds, or toasted coconut can add flavor and crunch to meals, mimicking the texture of nuts in salads or granola.
- ***Nut-Free Flours:*** Almond or cashew flours are often used in gluten-free baking. For nut-free alternatives, ingredients such as oat flour, coconut flour, or chickpea flour provide comparable options.

- *Spreads and Butter:* Nut-free spreads like sunflower seed butter or soy-based butter are available to replace peanut or almond butter in recipes. These alternatives retain the creamy texture and use nut-based spreads without including allergens.
- *Nut-Free Garnishes:* For garnishes or toppings, seeds such as flax, sesame, or sunflower seeds may be used in place of nuts, depending on individual dietary needs.

When preparing nut-free recipes, it is important to ensure cooking surfaces, utensils, and equipment are free of nut residues to avoid cross-contamination.

Nutrition Considerations & Substitutes

Nuts are valued for their nutritional contributions, including healthy fats, protein, fiber, vitamins, and minerals. On a nut-free diet, alternative sources of these nutrients can be incorporated.

- *Healthy Fats:* Nut-free options such as avocado, fish, seeds, olive oil, and coconut oil provide unsaturated fats for heart health.
- *Protein:* Beans, lentils, legumes, and soy products offer plant-based protein options. Animal-derived proteins from meat, eggs, and dairy are also nut-free sources.

- *Fiber:* Fruits, vegetables, whole grains, and legumes are rich sources of fiber and can fill the gap left by excluding nuts from the diet.
- *Vitamins and Minerals:* Seeds, leafy greens, dairy products, and fortified cereals can provide key micronutrients like magnesium, zinc, and vitamin E, which are commonly found in nuts.

By considering these nutritional substitutes, individuals can maintain a balanced diet without the inclusion of nuts. Identifying nut-free variations of commonly used ingredients and understanding dietary alternatives ensures that nutritional needs are met while adhering to a nut-free lifestyle.

Nut-Free Sample Recipes

Eating well with a nut allergy doesn't mean sacrificing variety or flavor. Below are a selection of nut-free recipes for breakfast, lunch, dinner, snacks, and desserts. These dishes are crafted with safe ingredients, ensuring they are suitable for individuals with nut allergies.

Breakfast

Oat-Free Energy Bowl

This bowl is packed with energy without the use of oats or nuts, making it both allergy-safe and delicious.

Ingredients:

- 1 cup cooked quinoa, chilled
- 1/2 cup dairy-free yogurt (or traditional yogurt, if preferred)
- 1 banana, sliced
- 1/2 cup fresh berries (strawberries, blueberries, or raspberries)
- 1 tablespoon chia seeds
- 1 tablespoon sunflower seeds (optional, ensure they are nut-contamination free)
- 1/2 teaspoon honey or maple syrup for sweetness (optional)

Instructions:

1. Start by placing the chilled quinoa at the bottom of your bowl.
2. Add a layer of yogurt over the quinoa.
3. Arrange the banana slices and berries on top.
4. Sprinkle chia seeds and sunflower seeds over the fruit.
5. Drizzle honey or maple syrup for added sweetness if desired.

Nut-Free Granola

A crunchy granola without any risk of nuts, ideal for breakfast or snacking.

Ingredients:

- 3 cups puffed rice cereal or buckwheat groats
- 1 cup shredded coconut (unsweetened, nut-free approved)
- 1/2 cup pumpkin seeds
- 1/4 cup flaxseeds
- 1/4 cup dried fruit (raisins, cranberries, or apricots—check labels for added oils)
- 1/4 cup sunflower oil or melted coconut oil
- 1/4 cup honey or maple syrup
- 1 teaspoon vanilla extract

Instructions:

1. Set your oven to 350°F (175°C) and prepare a baking sheet by lining it with parchment paper.
2. Mix the puffed rice, shredded coconut, pumpkin seeds, flaxseeds, and dried fruit in a large bowl.
3. Combine the oil, honey or maple syrup, and vanilla extract, then pour over the dry ingredients. Mix thoroughly.

4. Spread the granola mixture evenly over the baking sheet.
5. Bake for 15–20 minutes, stirring halfway to ensure even browning.
6. Cool completely before storing in an airtight container.

Sweet Potato Hash with Eggs

Ingredients:

- 1 medium sweet potato, diced
- 1/2 bell pepper, diced
- 1/2 onion, chopped
- 2 tablespoons olive oil
- 2 eggs
- Salt and pepper to taste

Instruction:

1. In a large skillet, heat 2 tablespoons of olive oil over medium-high heat.
2. Add the diced sweet potato, bell pepper, and onion to the skillet and cook until tender, about 10 minutes.
3. Crack two eggs into the skillet on top of the cooked vegetables.
4. Season with salt and pepper to taste.
5. Cover the skillet and let it cook for an additional 3-5 minutes until the eggs are cooked to your desired consistency.
6. Serve hot as a delicious and filling breakfast option.

Nut-Free Smoothie

Ingredients:

- 1 cup almond-free milk (e.g., rice milk)
- 1 frozen banana
- 1/2 cup frozen strawberries
- 1 tablespoon sunflower seed butter

Instructions:

1. Add all ingredients to a blender.
2. Blend until smooth and creamy.
3. Serve immediately for a refreshing and nutritious breakfast option.
4. Optional: top with additional sliced fruit or a sprinkle of hemp seeds for added texture and flavor.

Coconut Chia Pudding

Ingredients:

- 1/2 cup coconut milk
- 2 tablespoons chia seeds
- 1/2 teaspoon vanilla extract
- Fruit toppings (e.g., mango, berries)

Instructions:

1. In a small bowl, mix together the coconut milk, chia seeds, and vanilla extract.
2. Cover and refrigerate for at least 4 hours or overnight, until the mixture becomes thick and pudding-like.
3. Top with fresh fruit before serving for a delicious and nutrient-rich breakfast option.
4. Tip: Add in other toppings such as nuts or shredded coconut for added flavor and texture.

Lunch & Dinner

Allergy-Friendly Stir-Fry

This stir-fry is a quick and flavorful nut-free meal packed with colorful vegetables.

Ingredients:

- 2 tablespoons sunflower oil (or any safe cooking oil)
- 1 chicken breast, thinly sliced, or firm tofu cubes for a vegetarian option
- 1 cup broccoli florets
- 1 red bell pepper, thinly sliced
- 1 medium carrot, julienned
- 1/2 cup snap peas
- 2 cloves garlic, minced
- 1 teaspoon grated fresh ginger
- 3 tablespoons soy sauce or tamari (ensure nut-free)
- 1 teaspoon cornstarch mixed with 2 tablespoons water

Instructions:

1. Heat the oil in a large pan or wok over medium-high heat. Add the chicken or tofu and cook until golden. Remove and set aside.
2. Add the vegetables to the pan and stir-fry for 5–7 minutes until tender-crisp.

3. Add the garlic and ginger, cooking for an additional 1 minute.
4. Return the chicken or tofu to the pan. Add the soy sauce and cornstarch mixture, stirring until the sauce thickens.
5. Serve immediately with steamed rice or noodles.

Chicken & Veggie Wraps

Ingredients:

- 2 large nut-free tortillas
- 1 cup shredded cooked chicken breast
- 1/2 cup diced cucumber
- 1/2 cup shredded carrots
- 1/4 cup shredded lettuce
- 2 tablespoons sunflower seed butter (optional, as a spread)
- 1 tablespoon lemon juice

Instructions:

1. Lay the tortillas flat. Spread sunflower seed butter thinly across the center (optional).
2. Layer the chicken, cucumber, carrots, and lettuce on top.
3. Drizzle with lemon juice for added freshness.
4. Roll the tortillas tightly into wraps, tucking the edges as you go. Cut in half before serving.

Lentil & Quinoa Salad

Ingredients:

- 1 cup cooked quinoa
- 1/2 cup cooked lentils
- 1/2 cucumber, diced
- 1/4 cup diced tomato
- 2 tablespoons olive oil
- Lemon juice to taste

Instructions:

1. In a large bowl, combine the cooked quinoa and lentils.
2. Add in the diced cucumber and tomato.
3. Drizzle with olive oil and lemon juice to taste.
4. Toss to combine all ingredients evenly.
5. Serve as a healthy and protein-packed side dish or main course salad.

Potato & Leek Soup

Ingredients:

- 3 potatoes, diced
- 2 leeks, sliced
- 4 cups nut-free vegetable broth
- 1 tablespoon olive oil

Instructions:

1. In a large pot, heat olive oil over medium-high heat.
2. Add in the diced potatoes and sliced leeks, sautéing for 5 minutes until slightly softened.
3. Pour in the vegetable broth and bring to a boil.
4. Reduce heat to low and let simmer for 20 minutes or until potatoes are tender.
5. Using an immersion blender or transfer small batches to a blender, puree the soup until smooth.
6. Serve hot with a sprinkle of fresh herbs on top (optional).

Turkey Meatballs with Rice

Ingredients:

- 1 lb ground turkey
- 1 egg
- 1/4 cup breadcrumbs
- 2 cups cooked rice

Instructions:

1. Heat the oven to 375°F (190°C) and line a baking tray with parchment paper.
2. In a large bowl, mix together the ground turkey, egg, and breadcrumbs until well combined.
3. Roll the mixture into small balls and place them on the lined baking sheet.
4. Bake for 20-25 minutes or until meatballs are cooked through and lightly browned.
5. In a separate pot, prepare 2 cups of rice according to package instructions.
6. Serve the turkey meatballs over a bed of rice for a satisfying and easy dinner option.

Snacks & Desserts

Sunflower Seed Butter Cookies

Ingredients:

- 1/2 cup sunflower seed butter
- 1/2 cup sugar
- 1 egg
- 1 teaspoon vanilla extract

Instructions:

1. Set your oven to 350°F (175°C) and prepare a baking sheet by lining it with parchment paper.
2. Mix all the ingredients in a bowl until well combined.
3. Roll the dough into 1-inch balls and place them on the baking sheet. Gently flatten with a fork.
4. Bake for 8–10 minutes. Allow the cookies to cool on the sheet before serving.

Coconut Rice Pudding

Ingredients:

- 3/4 cup white rice (short-grain preferred)
- 2 cups coconut milk (ensure nut-free processing)
- 1 cup water
- 1/3 cup sugar (or to taste)
- 1/2 teaspoon vanilla extract
- 1/4 teaspoon cinnamon (optional)

Instructions:

1. Combine the rice, coconut milk, and water in a saucepan. Bring to a boil, then reduce to a simmer.
2. Stir frequently to prevent sticking and cook until the rice is tender (about 20 minutes).
3. Once the mixture thickens, remove from heat and stir in sugar, vanilla extract, and cinnamon.
4. Allow the pudding to cool slightly before serving warm, or chill for a cool dessert.

Apple Chips

Ingredients:

- 2 apples, thinly sliced
- 1 teaspoon cinnamon

Instructions:

1. Set your oven to 200°F (95°C) and prepare a baking sheet with parchment paper.
2. Arrange the apple slices on the baking sheet in a single layer.
3. Sprinkle cinnamon evenly over the apple slices.
4. Bake for 1 hour, then flip the apple slices and bake for an additional 1-2 hours until crispy.
5. Allow the chips to cool before serving or storing them in an airtight container for up to a week.

Frozen Yogurt Bark

Ingredients:

- 1 cup nut-free yogurt
- 1/4 cup diced strawberries
- 1/4 cup blueberries
- Optional: sprinkle of seeds or shredded coconut

Instructions:

1. Line a baking sheet with parchment paper.
2. Spread the yogurt evenly on the baking sheet, about 1/4 inch thick.
3. Top with diced strawberries, blueberries, and any optional toppings.
4. Freeze for at least 2 hours before breaking into pieces to serve.
5. Store in an airtight container in the freezer for up to 2-3 weeks.

Dairy-Free Chocolate Mousse

Ingredients:

- 1 cup coconut cream
- 1/4 cup cocoa powder
- 2 tablespoons sugar

Instructions:

1. In a mixing bowl, whip the coconut cream until it forms stiff peaks.
2. Gently fold in cocoa powder and sugar until well combined.
3. Spoon into individual serving dishes and chill for at least 2 hours before serving.
4. Garnish with toppings like fresh fruit or shaved chocolate if desired.
5. This rich and creamy chocolate mousse is a delicious dairy-free alternative to traditional mousse made with heavy cream.
6. These recipes demonstrate that nut-free cooking can be both exciting and delicious. By using safe, alternative ingredients, there's no shortage of options for those avoiding nuts in their meals.

Nut Allergies in Children & Social Settings

Children with nut allergies face unique challenges, particularly in social environments such as schools, daycare facilities, and group activities. Addressing these challenges requires awareness, clear communication, and thoughtful preparation to create a safe and inclusive environment.

Below, we explore key considerations in schools and daycare settings, communicating effectively with caregivers and friends, and navigating social situations involving anxiety.

Managing Allergies in Schools & Daycare

For children with nut allergies, schools, and daycare centers are critical areas where safety measures must be carefully implemented. Collaboration between families and school staff ensures that precautions are followed consistently.

- *Policies and Training:* Schools and daycare centers implement policies like nut-free zones and staff training to manage and respond to food allergies effectively.

- ***Emergency Action Plans:*** Written allergy action plans are commonly shared with schools or daycare facilities. These plans outline the child's specific allergens, symptoms of an allergic reaction, and step-by-step instructions for emergency response, including the use of an epinephrine auto-injector.
- ***Safe Lunches and Snacks:*** Families can pack allergen-free lunches, and schools may set guidelines to avoid foods that pose allergy risks.
- ***Classroom Activities:*** Teachers can reduce allergy risks by using safe substitutes for nut-based ingredients during food activities and opting for non-food rewards.
- ***Understanding Cross-Contamination:*** Educating staff and peers about cross-contamination risks—such as shared utensils, lunch tables, or surfaces—can help reduce accidental exposure.

The implementation of these safety measures contributes to maintaining a positive and controlled environment for children with nut allergies.

Communicating with Caregivers & Friends

Clear and effective communication is essential to protect children with nut allergies, particularly when they are under the care of individuals outside their families. Caregivers and friends can play a crucial role in maintaining safety when they have access to necessary information.

- *Explaining the Allergy:* Caregivers, babysitters, and other temporary guardians can be informed about the specific nature and severity of the child's allergy. Families may detail which foods, ingredients, or situations to avoid, and share information about recognizing allergic reactions.
- *Access to Emergency Plans:* Caregivers should be familiar with the child's emergency plan, including how to administer an epinephrine auto-injector. Providing resources or visual guides can aid their understanding.
- *Fostering Understanding Among Peers:* Friends and their families can benefit from learning how to manage social interactions safely. For instance, they can be encouraged to ask questions, learn which snacks are safe to share, or ensure their hands are clean after eating.

These conversations build trust and awareness, allowing individuals involved in the child's life to better understand their role in promoting safety.

Handling Social Situations & Anxiety

Participating in social situations, such as birthday parties, school trips, or community events, can bring concerns about potential allergen exposure. These situations require planning to minimize risks and address related anxieties in children.

- ***Ensuring a Supportive Environment:*** Hosted events, such as birthday parties or holiday celebrations, may include conversations with hosts about allergy-safe food options or arrangements. Providing the child's own allergen-free snacks can also reduce anxieties surrounding meals or treats.
- ***Encouraging Self-Advocacy:*** Depending on their age, children may learn to identify safe and unsafe foods, ask adults clarifying questions about ingredients, or carry their emergency medication.
- ***Managing Emotional Impact:*** Children with nut allergies may experience feelings of exclusion or heightened anxiety when interacting in group settings. Support from parents, teachers, or peers can alleviate some of this emotional stress. Tools such as mindfulness exercises or stress management strategies may help children remain confident and focused when navigating social environments.
- ***Building Peer Awareness:*** Positive interactions with peers can also foster empathy and inclusion. Peers who understand allergy concerns may be more likely to offer support during shared activities or meals.

Addressing both physical and emotional aspects of allergy management in social settings ensures that children feel safe and included while actively participating in everyday experiences.

By implementing preventative measures in schools and daycare facilities, establishing clear and open forms of communication, and preparing for social interactions, children with nut allergies can enjoy safer and more inclusive environments. Awareness and education are vital for fostering understanding and collaboration in these contexts.

Conclusion

Living with or caring for someone with a nut allergy can feel overwhelming, but you've taken an important step by educating yourself through this guide. Thank you for reading and equipping yourself with the knowledge necessary to better understand, manage, and prevent allergic reactions. Awareness and preparation are your strongest tools in safeguarding yourself or a loved one, and this guide has laid out practical steps to make life more manageable.

You now know the science behind nut allergies, the risks of cross-contamination, and how to recognize symptoms, whether mild or severe. Armed with this knowledge, you can take the lead in creating safe environments—whether at home, in schools, or social settings. By reading food labels carefully, communicating openly with caregivers and peers, and preparing for emergencies, you're not only reducing risks but also helping normalize the conversation around allergies, making it easier for others to join in your efforts.

While nut allergies require vigilance, this condition doesn't have to define your or anyone else's life. With early planning, clear communication, and confidence in managing risks, you or your loved one can enjoy celebrations, travel, and daily activities without constant fear. It's about finding what works best for your situation and empowering yourself to create positive and safe experiences.

Remember, every decision you make to stay informed, speak up, and plan ahead contributes to building a more inclusive environment for those affected by nut allergies. Your dedication fosters understanding and change, making the world a little safer—and a lot kinder—for everyone. Keep taking proactive steps, stay prepared, and know that you are not alone in this.

FAQs

What are the most common symptoms of a nut allergy?

Nut allergy symptoms can range from mild to severe. Mild symptoms include itching, hives, or swelling around the mouth and throat. Severe reactions, such as difficulty breathing, a rapid drop in blood pressure, or anaphylaxis, require immediate medical attention.

How can I know if I or my child has a nut allergy?

If you suspect a nut allergy, consult an allergist for testing. Common diagnostic methods include skin prick tests, blood tests, or an oral food challenge in a controlled medical environment. Proper diagnosis is crucial to manage the allergy effectively.

What is cross-contamination, and how can I avoid it?

Cross-contamination occurs when nut allergens come into contact with nut-free foods, often through shared utensils, surfaces, or cooking equipment. To avoid it, use separate utensils and cookware for nut-free meals, clean surfaces thoroughly, and check the packaging for warnings like "may contain nuts."

Can nut allergies develop later in life?

Yes, nut allergies can develop at any age, even if you've previously consumed nuts without issues. Factors like immune system changes or cross-reactivity with other allergens may contribute. If you experience allergic reactions, consult a doctor.

What should I do in case of an anaphylactic reaction?

Administer an epinephrine auto-injector immediately and call emergency services. While waiting for medical help, monitor the person and help keep them calm. Do not delay using epinephrine if severe symptoms appear.

How can I ensure my food is nut-free when dining out?

Notify restaurant staff of your allergy and ask specific questions about ingredients and preparation. Avoid dishes with unclear ingredient lists or those prepared in shared fryers or cooking spaces, as they may pose risks of cross-contact.

What are safe alternatives to nuts for snacks or cooking?

Safe alternatives include seeds like sunflower or pumpkin seeds, coconut, roasted chickpeas, and nut-free spreads such as sunflower seed butter. Always check labels to ensure they are processed in nut-free environments.

References and Helpful Links

Weiss, K. (2024, April 23). Your guide to peanut and nut allergies. Healthline.
https://www.healthline.com/health/allergies/nut-allergy-symptoms

Nut allergies. (n.d.). Mount Sinai Health System.
https://www.mountsinai.org/health-library/diseases-conditions/nut-allergies

Avoiding cross-contamination - Food Allergy Canada. (2021, January 15). Food Allergy Canada.
https://foodallergycanada.ca/living-with-allergies/day-to-day-management/avoiding-cross-contamination/

Recipe substitutions for peanut or nut allergy. (2023, January 13). Kids With Food Allergies.
https://kidswithfoodallergies.org/recipes-diet/recipe-substitutions/substitutions-for-peanuts-and-tree-nuts/

Huffstetler, E. (2019, August 12). 7 ingredients you can use as a nut substitute. The Spruce Eats.
https://www.thespruceeats.com/baked-goods-nut-substitutes-1388892

Hummusapien. (n.d.). Easy, healthy nut free recipes - Hummusapien.
https://www.hummusapien.com/recipes/diet/nut-free/

Kids Health Info : Peanut and tree nut allergy. (n.d.). https://www.rch.org.au/kidsinfo/fact_sheets/Peanut_and_tree_nut_allergy/

Tree Nut | Causes, Symptoms & Treatment | ACAAI Public Website. (2024, January 23). ACAAI Patient. https://acaai.org/allergies/allergic-conditions/food/tree-nut/

Allergy & Asthma Associates & Allergy & Asthma Associates. (2017, June 6). 11 Tasty Recipes for Children with Nut Allergies - Allergy and Asthma Associates, S.C. Allergy and Asthma Associates, S.C. https://foxcitiesallergists.com/11-tasty-recipes-for-children-with-nut-allergies/

www.ingramcontent.com/pod-product-compliance
Lightning Source LLC
LaVergne TN
LVHW012031060526
838201LV00061B/4560